MW01289300

The Psychology of Finally Being

Full From Within

Dr. Colleen Long, Psy.D.

"The secret of change is to focus all of your energy not on fighting the old, but on building the new."

- Socrates

Stay Looped In:

Website: SchoolofSelfHelp.com

Full From Within Course: SchoolofSelfHelp.Teachable.com

Email: talkdoc@DrColleenLong.com

Twitter: @TalkDoc

Youtube: Dr. Colleen Long

Instagram: @DrColleenLong

Facebook: facebook.com/DrColleen (friend request and message to be added to private support community)

Table of Contents

Acknowledgements

Thank you to all the thousands of patients who've allowed me to bear witness to the incredible power of the human will to change and evolve.

Thank you to my three toddlers for sacrificing some of our play time so mommy could "do her."

Thank you to my incredible husband who didn't bat an eye when I told him I was going to write this book.

To the Reader

At this point, you have probably gained and lost hundreds of pounds, but may have found in all of your attempts- they only focused on what type of foods to eat vs. helping you understand why you overeat in the first place.

This psychological aspect of weight loss is fundamental if one is to truly sustain change vs. doing yet another diet. This book will provide you with real life practical behavioral tools to avoid common maladaptive eating patterns (emotional eating, bingeing, food addiction, etc).

Another vital component to this book is the private online support available through our Facebook page:

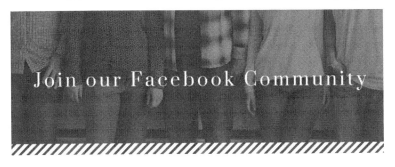

http://www.facebook.com/drcolleen

If you are interested in being added, please send a friend request to the above link, and message me that you would like to be added to the group.

Why Do I Need a Support Group?

The two pillars in all addiction recovery are interpersonal relationships and spirituality. Through our online support community, you can ask questions maybe you've been too embarrassed to ask your surgeon or friends. You can share trials and tribulations along your weight loss journey. One of the major reasons a support group is so important in any major change is that it makes it feel more "real." How many times have you started a diet on Monday, only to revert back to bad habits by Friday?

I truly hope that this is a valuable component of your weight loss journey. Enjoy!

Dr. Colleen

Welcome to
a Modern Way
of Relating
to Food

Welcome and thank you for taking yet another step towards ensuring your personal and sustained weight loss success. I have been working in the field of weight loss surgery since 2009. I have probably spoke with over 1000 people who struggle with obesity by now.

The universal truth is that all of these people realized the consciousness that got them into the problem (being overweight or morbid obesity), wasn't going to be the only thing capable of solving it. They understood that they needed outside help, a power tool, to really lose the weight for good- for the last time.

Unfortunately, I didn't see many patients post-operatively. They usually were successful with the sleeve or bypass, felt better about themselves, isolated less, exercised more- and so in turn, many of their psychological symptoms went away.

However, as I delved further into the online world of support for vsg and wls, I learned it wasn't all rainbows and butterflies. Many people might have breezed through the honeymoon phase of their weight loss surgery (first 6 months- 1 year), but then started to gain the weight back.

The honeymoon phase is easy: it consists of an initial phase of liquids, where there is no gray area, no room for trouble. Then a slight adjustment into re-introducing semi solids, and then re-adapting to life on life's terms, but with a much healthier approach to food.

At the outset, people lose most of their weight within this first year period and feel the most powerful sense of efficacy they have felt in a while. They are getting social feedback that is extremely reinforcing and makes getting through the cravings and urges a bit easier.

However, as time passes. When everyone goes home from the party- and that honeymoon phase is over- the person is still left with many of their demons that got them overweight in the first place.

Perhaps they had trauma and used weight as a buffer or cushion from the outside world. Maybe they turned to food for nurturance when they grieved the loss of their mother or father. Maybe they used food mindlessly when they were with their kids, or grazed throughout the day in a job that burnt them out mentally.

Whatever the psychological factors were that contributed to the problem, were often over shadowed in the post-op glow of weight loss surgery.

Yet, as I started to see more and more people come into my practice 2 and 3 years post, or even just looked at the dialogue on the chat boards, I knew something still needed to be addressed.

People still failed to address the "why," and instead only had been focusing on the "what," of food.

By the time they realized this- it was usually two years post and they were too embarrassed to come in and say "hey I need help." Unfortunately, I would see all too often, people waiting to come back in until things got their worst, and then needing a sleeve to bypass conversion.

I realized the common thread was humiliation. Because

we can't put our thumb on psychological factors, we often don't give them the same importance that we give Hypertension, Diabetes, or Sleep Apnea. There is no blood test for Depression.

However, the psychological component to obesity is the silent monster lurking in the shadows, waiting to re-emerge when all the shininess wears off.

Enter- Full From Within.

The Honeymoon is over.

If you are reading this book, it is likely that you have experienced some success now with weight loss surgery, but are craving additional motivation and inspiration. Maybe you are noticing that your weight loss is plateauing or worse- starting to creep back.

You might be realizing now the psychological demons you faced before are starting to resurface and that they must finally be dealt with if you are to truly maintain your weight loss for a lifetime.

You might also just be a really proactive person who is only considering weight loss surgery and want to feel fully informed before just diving in head first. For that, I congratulate you.

In whatever case, it is important to know that weight loss surgery is not a magic bullet, a magic wand, or even "cheating." Procedures like gastric sleeve, bypass, and balloon are merely power tools in helping one achieve their goals whilst simultaneously putting in place all the other things one needs to do to lose weight and become healthier (not overeating, reducing portion sizes, planning for meals, eating healthier food, using food only for physiological hunger, exercising, reducing sweets and carbs, etc.)

The darker more insidious piece that keeps most people in the grips of food addiction, is often not discussed in the weight loss surgery world. A world where we want to believe that with a relatively short procedure, we can "cut out" our demons.

There is a much more complex piece to food addiction and all addictions in general- our deeply held unconscious belief system and a malfunctioning reward/pleasure system.

This book's goal is to help shed light on this darker piece that often gets people stuck. If the book feels repetitive, it is for a reason. This book is divided into two major sections: *clearing out the old*- where we bring to the surface the thoughts, feelings, and behaviors that have contributed to our obesity, and *bringing in the new*- which is going to help you begin to cultivate a happier self and a healthier relationship to food. By cultivating this new way of living, you will begin to understand what it means to be truly full from within.

Additionally, there are "mind meals" at the end of each chapter that challenge you to think critically about how these principles uniquely apply to you. This is the glue of this book.

The other major piece of this book is that it parallels my own work with patients in private practice. I have found, for them to successfully make such a monumental change with their relationship to food, there must be a highly structured approach. This book provides you with the framework I use everyday, but it is up to you to uniquely format it to your own interests, thoughts, and desires.

We can all understand information on a conceptual basis, but actually taking the time to think about how those concepts apply in our life is the piece that will finally allow us to feel from within.

As you read, try to let the layer of guilt and self-loathing that you've carried for so long melt away. It doesn't serve you and in fact- probably perpetuates the problem. Understand that we can all become conditioned to want the wrong things, despite our most intelligent processes.

Finally, allow yourself to relax and be open to the new information this book will present to your unconscious mind.

Chapter 1

What Does it Mean to be Truly Full From Within?

Oftentimes, when I would interview a pre-op weight loss surgery patient- they would say "I never seem to feel full, I feel like I could always eat more." Something I started to realize over time was that, for many, the term "full," meant more than just being satisfied from hunger. It meant feeling distracted, numb, feeling less, feeling more. Food, for so many has taken on way more meaning than its simple purpose- to fuel us to survive.

I recognized that if people were ever to feel truly full, it would mean looking at what they were trying to fill up, psychologically. For some, they have insight right away, "whenever I have to deal with my mother-in-law, I have to have a bag of chips by my nightstand," or "whenever a stressful meeting is coming up, I know I will be crunching away on something right before."

However, for many- the internal "black hole," doesn't surface until after the surgery. One lady came in to therapy afterwards and said "I didn't realize how lonely I am in a house full of people." Food was her companion and she was grieving its loss.

In this book, I will try to help guide you to go within and think about your own internal black hole. Most of us have them, it is just that different people try to fill it with different things; money, sex, drugs, alcohol, relationships, food.

You have simply conditioned your brain to be reinforced by food. The rule of the brain is that what fires together, wires together. If you pair stress with eating food over time- you create a strongly reinforced reward system, whereby food becomes a powerful mechanism to give you relaxation.

Yet over time, it isn't really the food that provides the stress relief- *it is the freedom from the wanting.* [11] In other words, it is not food that provides you with enjoyment, but relief from the discomfort of wanting.

What if we could cure ourselves from wanting food for all the wrong reasons? In OA there is a saying "with drug and alcohol addiction recovery, you slay the dragon, but with food addiction recovery- you have to take it out for a walk three times a day."

What if your "dragon" no longer held the same meaning? What if this whole process wasn't a sad and scary time of letting go of a long-time friend, but an exhilarating and optimistic time of ushering in a new life? Another chance at being the person you always knew was there under the surface?

Full From Within aims to equip you with the psychological tools to fundamentally shift your way of relating to food. If we shed light on our psychological "holes," and fill them up in the right ways- we will never white knuckle a diet again.

Mind Meal : Can you think of something else in your life that you have "slayed?" What behaviors worked? What thoughts worked? What rules did you implement to ensure success? Can you think of how your past success could apply to your relationship with food?

_____

_____

_____

_____

_____

_____

_____

Chapter 2

Do I need a Shrink?

I see the road to recovery from any addiction in three levels; psychological, fulfillment, and behavioral. The psychological level (level 1) being the most severe and behavioral level (level 3) being more mild. Another way to visualize these levels is to think of the ocean. There is the sand at the bottom of sea- and that is where you are if you are struggling with untreated mental health issues.

If you are not struggling with mental health issues, but are unhappy, discontent, and unfulfilled psychologically, then you may not be stuck in the sand, but you are still underwater- unable to grasp the help that is waiting for you above water.

Lastly, if you are happy and content most of the time, but realize you have some long reinforced behaviors that need to be nipped in the bud, your head is above water and you are in the best place possible to receive, retain, and retrain the brain with this information.

This book is written for levels two and three. Full From Within is designed to provide people with the factors they need to cultivate internal psychological fulfillment, creating healthier ways of relating to food, as well as stopping old bad habits and creating newer healthier alternatives.

Level One

At level one- there are people who truly suffer with psychologically diagnosable conditions such as Bipolar Disorder, Major Depressive Disorder, Generalized Anxiety Disorder, Etc. They might also have experienced other addictions in the past to drugs and alcohol, or physical and sexual trauma. When I encounter these individuals during a pre-operative evaluation, I always refer them out for treatment first, because they are less likely to be successful in the long term.

Think about it- if they are unable to even get out of bed in the morning because they have debilitating depression, how likely are they going to be to sustain an exercise regimen, or much less- attend follow up appointments?

Below are key hallmark signs that you may suffer from a diagnosable condition and likely need to seek professional help while embarking on your weight loss journey:

- feeling of internal "heaviness," or "sadness," for no reason

- feeling of impending doom, something bad about to happen

- feeling of panic, anxiety coming out of nowhere

- feeling less interested in the things that once interested you

- Isolating vs. socializing (not just due to your weight)

- decreased libido

- impulsive/compulsive behaviors in addition to bingeing (gambling, shopping, drinking, etc)

- feeling worse in the morning

- having difficulty getting started in the morning

- intermittent bouts of tearfulness

- excessive or inappropriate anger

- saying something or doing something and then later regretting it

If you answered yes to four or more of the above items, you should seek professional help before attempting your weight loss program. You can visit psychologytoday.com or goodtherapy.org, click on "find a therapist," and type in your zip code and find therapists in your area. A great feature of these websites is the ability to filter by insurance and even specialty.

If you have not yet had the surgery, I strongly encourage you to have at least six weeks of treatment under your belt before undergoing the procedure.

Level Two

The next level is that of fulfillment. This is for the people who don't necessarily have depression or other diagnosable psychiatric symptoms, but just feel disenchanted or discontent with life. They feel like "is this all there is?" and oftentimes will feel like they are in a life rut.

This next level is equally important because if we are unfulfilled, we often will use "things" to try to fill ourselves up. Hence the name "Full From Within." It is upon us to create the internal psychological structure to no longer need external "filling up."

In my book, Happiness in B.A.L.A.N.C.E- What We Know Now (2010)[18], I discuss the seven researched principles of fulfillment, based on the research.

It is important to assess whether or not we have all of these factors in place before starting our weight loss journey. If we are psychologically running on "E" then recovery from food addiction or attachment will be an uphill battle. But if we are truly *full from within*, food loses its power.

Level Three

This level comprises the behavioral issues that get one into trouble when it comes to weight. They usually don't report that they eat for emotional reasons, but that the biggest contributing factor to their weight is in the portion sizes they consume, the types of food they eat, and the failure to plan.

Usually, people in the level three category tend to experience success more readily than the first two levels simply because they have less they have to address in terms of the psychological.

I find that many of these people are members of the "clean plate club," and simple cognitive reframes such as "would you rather the food waste in the waste basket or on your waist?" can go a long way in helping them change.

In fact, the group of people who's single problem is the fact they clean their plate at every setting and in general, eat too large of portion sizes, are the people who tend to have the easiest time with this surgery. In my experience over the last 9 years, this group tends to be largely comprised of men.

The second factor in this level are those that have poor nutritional habits; carb lovers, sugar addicts, processed food, etc. The nutritionist is usually the most helpful professional for this group of people in that they can provide healthier alternatives for whatever has been getting them into trouble.

The last part of level three are those that don't think about food until it is too late, often consuming most of their daily calories between 6 and 10 pm (or the last part of their day if they work the night shift).

The saying "if you fail to plan, plan to fail," comes to mind for this subtype. For many, it seems counterintuitive to think about food *more* to weigh *less*. However, people that tend to meal prep, naturally have more success with eating healthier throughout the week because they decrease the amount of "grey area" that gets us all into trouble.

Think about it, you've skipped breakfast because you rushed out the door to work, you worked past lunch because you had a deadline to meet, and now it is 3 pm and you're ravenous. Are you going to grab a salad, or go for a heavy sandwich or pasta dish at this point?

We will go more into the solutions for this subtype later in the book. But know that this level is the most easily "fixable" level when it comes to weight loss. The bad habits are less embedded in our psyche and more about simple behavioral change.

This book is built in two parts. One part is aimed at helping the "level 3's" understand why maladaptive eating patterns are so hard to break in the first place and then providing the guidance as to how to clip those old wires and develop new behavioral pathways.

The second part of this book is aimed at helping the "level 2's" who's needs may extend beyond the behavioral. If you are a level 2 you realize you need to first work on getting your head above water by finding inner contentment and THEN work on changing your eating patterns. This book will help give you those tools.

Lastly, the first half of this book is aimed at "clearing out the old," and the second half is about "filling you back up." Given the title of this book- my aim is to first help you clear out the toxicity from a previous maladaptive relationship with food. When you build a house, you can't just build a new foundation on top of an unstable one. You must first clear out the old to make way for the new. Same thing any farmer knows about cultivating a good harvest. You have to kill the weeds to make room for bountiful growth.

This is exactly what this book aims to do. The first part will be hitting at many of the toxic "weeds" that get people into trouble in the first place. The second half will then provide the "filling up" part. In my opinion, this is the most frequently missed part in so many self-help books.

So many books tell us what NOT to do, but then leave us with a "white-knuckle" mentality at the end. We are left to just sit in our life and tell ourselves over and over again not to do the very thing that we have conditioned ourselves to do for so long. This book provides you with real life, practical tools to cultivate joy and create a new way of defining quality of life.

Mind Meal: Do you consider yourself a level 1, 2, or 3? What factors lead you to believe you are this level?

_____

_____

_____

_____

_____

_____

_____

Clearing
Out
the Old

Chapter 3

Doing the real work

" The wound is where the light enters you."

- Rumi

1 in every 8 Americans is on some form of psychotropic medications. [28] In his book, Anatomy of an Epidemic, science journalist Robert Whitaker states that since 1987, the percentage of the population receiving federal disability payment for mental illness has tripled; among children under the age of 18, the percentage has grown by a factor of 35. [28]

While he recognized that in the short-term, these medications help people to feel better, he started to realize that over time- drugs make many patients sicker than they would have been if they had never been medicated. [28]

He does not make the argument that all people should stop their meds. He believes in the utility of them, just more sparingly than they are currently utilized.

However, throughout my years in the practice of therapy- I have noticed a trend of moving people away from feeling. Crying is actually a symptom in the DSM-V. We have pathologized a human feeling!

When psychiatrists and therapists witness a patient tearful too many times in session, their next conclusion is that something must be wrong and they must be medicated.

This frustrates me so much as a clinician and as a person who has done her share of work in her own personal therapy. When we are broken, we are broken open. Being broken is a starting point, not a symptom that something has gone awry.

It is at the point of our deepest pain and grief that we have the greatest opportunity for growth. I find myself telling patients over and over- "you can't "get over" it, you must "go through" it."

Yet, so many of us have been indoctrinated to think that if we spend more than a day being sad, we must have depression, or if we feel nervous a little bit longer than we'd like to- we must have an anxiety disorder. We definitely "are Bipolar" if we have a mood swing.

We have been taught to not feel the yin, only the yang of our emotions. It's societally acceptable to talk about how happy your weekend was, or how much fun you had on vacation- but watch the uncomfortable shifting in chairs that takes place when you open up about how you just haven't felt like yourself lately.

In our world of quick fixes, where we can have a conference across the world, over a computer, communicate a message in two seconds via text, or post a picture that all of our family can see instantly- we also want instant relief for our suffering.

Yet, suffering is part of the human condition. It is through experiencing our deepest sorrows, we are able to appreciate our greatest joys. But we must first be willing to sit in the muck.

Part and parcel of any addiction (food, drugs, alcohol, etc.) is that the addict is particularly uncomfortable with being uncomfortable. However, the cure is right there for the taking.

"So what does this look like in real life?" you ask. "How do I open the wound and clear out the infection that started all of this in the first place?"

You start with presence. You start with a still and open heart. You start with a spiritual vulnerability that allows you to be at peace with not knowing what will happen next. You sit broken open and wait for the light to enter over time.

The most important piece in all of this is being able to create a consistent forum where you hold the space. This could be a therapist's office, it could be a weekly walk with a friend, a journal practice, or it could be as simple as a prayer every night.

You set the priority to hold the space and to sit in the muck. Maybe it starts with emotions that have no words? Maybe it starts with visceral, physical feelings, that you have to simply sit with for a while? Maybe you are lucky enough to immediately put in words where your wound all started and its just floating around in your thoughts, waiting to be articulated? Perhaps it starts with a behavior you tend to do all of the time that you know comes from a place of pain?

Case Study:

I had a client who continuously posted on social media sites. She had a constant need to feel recognized and admired. She knew there was something behind it and wanted to get to the bottom of where this was coming from.

Session over session, we sat with that need. We talked about what she wanted to get from each of those posts and why she was still "on E," left with an empty psychological tank.

The short story of Narcissus goes that he disdained people who loved him. After Nemesis noticed this he lured him to a pool that cast his own reflection. Narcissus fell in love with this pool, not realizing it was merely an image. Unable to leave the beauty of his reflection, he lost his will to live. He stared at this reflection until he died. [59]

Growing up, this client never quite got the love and admiration we all need from our parents. When we love something so much and don't get that back- it is that unrequited love that leaves a narcissistic wound. It doesn't necessarily always start with parents. It can be a formative romantic relationship, but it usually starts with parents.

When we are flying from couch to couch saying "look at me mommy I'm superman!" and our mom says "get off that couch now!" instead of "look at how strong and powerful you are," we begin forming the wound. Unfortunately, without recognizing this- many people will go throughout their life trying to heal it through other people or other things instead of within themselves. (recall the wizard of oz's moral of the story).

It was up to this client to stop the instinctual need to post and each time she had this inclination to look within for what she needed. Eventually, she developed a muscle for self validation, and the posting behavior stopped.

The lesson in this case study is to hopefully help guide you to your wound. If we have an addiction and feel out of control, you can bet we have a wound. Instead of distracting through bad habits, addictions, unhealthy relationships, or external wants- it is time to finally create a place of presence to start the healing process.

Mind Meal: Sit in silence for at least 15 minutes. Visualize in your mind's eye your heart with a bridge of white light to your head. What does it say? Where is the pain? Where is the wound? How might you start filling yourself up for good?

_____

_____

_____

_____

_____

_____

_____

Chapter 4

Melting the Iceberg

Studies show that we have two separate cognitive (thinking) systems- the conscious and the unconscious.[5] In more psychological terms, our brain can be looked at as two different parts, selves, or people. There is the conscious part of us that continues to engage in the bingeing and mindless eating, self loathes, and says "why do I continue to self sabotage? why do I keep doing something that I know is no longer working for me?"

But there is a glacial iceberg underneath the surface that is our unconscious mind, which has been programmed and inundated with societal messages about how food is good, how it helps us feel better, how it helps us feel less alone, secure, or energized.

Our unconscious tells us a story about why it would be a good idea to over eat and we believe it, because we don't know we have another choice.

Unconscious learning happens automatically and unintentionally through experiences, observations, conditioning and practice. [2] We begin to believe that food actually relaxes us, that it takes away our stress, that it nurtures us and makes us safe (all while ironically killing us when we over indulge in the long term). These things are deeply held beliefs below our conscious awareness and thus the reason we continue to gorge ourselves long after we realize the behavior is taking more than it gives.

A more neurological way to look at one's addiction to food is through different parts of our brain. Our most evolved brain- the frontal cortex tells us that we need to stop, that our eating is out of control, and in some cases- literally killing us.

However, our addicted midbrain (reptilian brain) has been calling the shots as a result of being positively reinforced for years. It continues to tell us a story about how we need whatever the chosen substance is (cigarettes, alcohol, food, etc). I repeat- our midbrain is in control, NOT our frontal better thinking cortex during the course of any addiction.[3]

This is why, despite most peoples' best intentions to change, they find it very hard to do so- because they aren't yet mindful enough of this process. Over time the reward center starts to take over and becomes dysfunctionally functional- which is what Kevin McCauley refers to as "pleasure unwoven," in his groundbreaking film on addiction.[4]

This process calls for repetitive neural **re**programming.

In this book, you will start this neural reprogramming because the content we are discussing will begin to challenge your unconscious and malfunctioning reward system to think differently about food and plant the necessary seeds of change.

"Anything unconscious dissolves when you shine the light of consciousness on it." -Eckhart Tolle

Mind Meal: What ideas and beliefs do you feel have long been ingrained in the way you relate to food? Are there certain cultural factors? things your parents told you about food (clean your plate, there are starving children in Africa, etc).

_____

_____

_____

_____

_____

_____

_____

full hypnosis videos to go along with this program can be found in the Full From Within Ultimate online course at SchoolofSelfHelp.Teachable.com

Chapter 5

The Ego & the Pain Body

To be able to truly understand what is at the core of our unhealthy attachment with food is to understand the ego and the pain body. So many people come in my office, trying to understand why they have one vision for themselves they want so badly, yet they just can't seem to get there.

Enter the Ego & the Pain Body.

The Ego is something we all have. In this context, I don't mean "ego" in the since that we are all narcissistic, more so that we all have built a part of ourselves that identifies with things. If we are truly attached or enmeshed with our ego, then we begin to not see the difference between ourselves and our ego.

If I am deeply attached to my ego- I might overly identify as a psychologist, or insist that people call me "doctor," in all settings (even though my husband still maintains I am not a "real doctor"). If I grew up believing I was highly intelligent,

I might become attached to this idea- and whenever challenged by any other seemingly intelligent individual, become fearful and angry.

Deepak Chopra refers to the Ego and standing for "edging god out." He and many others, see it as the part of us, self-created, that separates us from our original source.

However, you want to look at the concept of ego, for the purposes of this book just understand that it is something we all have and that the goal in our psychological evolution is to be able to see when it is in action, and not be controlled by it, to be detached from it, all the while, watching it clamor for attention like a child having a tantrum.

To begin to truly create change in our lives, we must first identify our own ego. What are we attached to? What people or concepts really drive us up a wall? Someone who is more gregarious (hey I'm supposed to be the social butterfly)? Someone who is more funny (I was always the class clown)? Someone who is more well read (I have always prided myself on being the most knowledgeable in the room). You get the idea.

Once we've identified what things our ego is tied to, it is our job to be able to watch it in action. For instance, if my ego is strongly attached to the concept that I am the smartest in the room, and someone commands attention at a dinner party because of their dynamic views on politics, I might try to one up them, or engage in a debate. However, if I know this about my ego- I might sit and feel the sting of not letting my ego do what it wants.

Our goal is to make our egos feel the sting of not doing what it wants all the time. Like an unruly child that has lacked years of discipline, we are going in and laying down the rules.

If my ego is fear based, then every time I encounter something that elicits fear- I might reach for a cookie or donut to satisfy and soothe my frightened ego. Yet, if I know my ego is fear based, I can sit with the fear and let my ego feel the sting instead of reaching for something externally.

Overtime, the more sting our ego feels, the more detached we become. The less controlled by our ego- we are, and the more connected to our original selves we are. When we feed the ego, we feed our depression and unhappiness. When we starve the ego, we feed our joy and self contentment.

The pain body is a derivative of the ego and a concept well discussed by Eckhart Tolle [9]. He sees it as the part of our selves that is the culmination of all the pain we have experienced thus far in our life.

If we are a sexual trauma survivor- our pain body will largely be composed of feelings of being out of control, victimized, controlled, and detached from our bodies. If we grew up with sad and depressed parents, our pain bodies are largely composed of sadness and looking at life as though the glass were half empty.

Tolle explains how strongly our pain body influences our daily behavior:

"It is not so much that you can't stop the train of negative thoughts produced by the pain body, but that you don't want to. This is because the pain body is living through you, pretending to be you, and to the pain body, pain is pleasure. It eagerly devours every negative thought. If it sounds to you like a psychic parasite- that is exactly what it is."

So what do we do about this psychic parasite? We expose it to the light of our conscious intention and attention. When we find ourselves mired in self defeat, helplessness, frustration, and negativity- we realize this is not us but the pain body parasite feasting away. We consciously set an intention to experience joy in that moment and find things in our environment to support that intention.

Overtime, after starving your parasite and exposing it to the light of your consciousness it will no longer survive. This is the goal in all significant change. We must truly look at the most inner layer of the human psyche and drive out the parasites.

Chapter 6

The Fundamental Shift

I have worked with gastric lapband, sleeve, bypass, and now balloon patients for over 9 years, and one concept I go over with them constantly is the fundamental shift that must take place before embarking on such a big change.

You can't just go into this thinking its another diet. You can't just white knuckle the problem and say "don't do it, don't do it, don't eat right now" over and over when you have a craving. You have to deeply change what you view as defining fun and quality of life.

For many patients who have weight issues, they have attached concepts beyond hunger satisfaction to food, including; stress relief, emotional comfort, nurturance, boredom relief, connection tool with family and friends, fatigue relief, the only justifiable break, sadness/emptiness relief, etc.

For someone to truly lose the weight for good, they must

be able to find alternative ways of getting those needs met. Unfortunately, the need for stress relief, nurturance, connection, and support don't go away after a major weight loss or weight loss surgery. Life is still there waiting for you, so you must figure out how you are going to meet those needs in a way that won't self sabotage.

I use the analogy of brushing one's teeth with food addicts. Because they have to eat food (unlike other addictions where one might just be able to stop cold turkey), they have to look at what they are doing as for fuel or health vs. enjoyment. When we brush our teeth we don't spend hours anticipating "where am I going to brush my teeth?" "what type of toothpaste will I use?" We just do it and move on. That is the way food has to shift in food addicts' mind.

Food is just something we do to fuel up, to maintain health. But, it is not the place we go to derive pleasure or happiness. We must be creative and find other ways to define quality of life.

Here's where I might lose you: An important step we must take in making this fundamental shift is *removing the pleasure from the eating experience*.

If we are eating an egg white omelette with veggies and Mrs. Dash in the morning, turkey on greens with light dressing for lunch, and a small piece of grilled chicken with broccoli for dinner- we will not likely come to look forward to our meals over time. This is exactly what we want.

If we have any expectation that we are going to derive pleasure from food- we let the devil in the door, as they say in the south. We open the opportunity for us to feel the need to throw in a little extra sauce, maybe some melted cheese, or even a small little bowl of noodles.

We have to rid our eating experiences of pleasure and re-condition ourselves to see it as fuel. Something that has been helpful for many in doing this, is immediately doing some pleasurable activity after the meal is over. 1) it encourages us to get done sooner and not draw the meal out, and 2) it reinforces to us that pleasure is found outside of eating.

Here are some examples of behaviors you can do immediately after eating:

- going for a walk in nature
- listening to music
- calling a friend
- having a tea ritual
- exercising
- buying a new pair of shoes, pants, etc
- getting a massage
- Playing with a child or a pet
- playing a game
- adult coloring book
- Organizing (if that is your thing)
- painting
- Writing
- going to see a movie in the middle of the day
- watching a funny you tube video
- making a photo flipagram or collage

You can have your own list of items that inspire you, but

the idea is to begin to reinforce to yourself that there are many other things waiting for you that will provide you with fun. Losing weight doesn't mean living a dull and unsatisfying life.

Mind Meal: Use the space below to write down some of your own pleasurable activities that don't involve food:

_____

_____

_____

_____

_____

_____

_____

Chapter 7

The Baptism

If you are reading this, you are likely on your 509th attempt at weight loss. You are frustrated and feel hopeless and alone. Maybe you finally feel differently because the prospect of gastric sleeve or bypass surgery has instilled new hope. In any event, looking back on all your attempts you can probably identify one concrete behavior that demarcated the beginning of all new diets.

It could have been "the last supper before,"... it could be one last party with all the yummy apps you love, it could be throwing out all your "fat clothes," it could be cleaning out your kitchen so that only healthy ingredients are left.

Whatever it is- you were doing something instinctively that needs to be done to help with success and true behavioral change. A baptism.

This time is no different. It is important to sit back and think about what you can do symbolically the moment before you plan to truly change your lifestyle forever.

Here are some examples that have worked for others:

throwing out all "trigger foods"

2) getting an expensive, luxurious container for water that signifies health and self care that will remind you to hydrate throughout the day

3) throwing out all your "fat clothes" so that there is only one way to go - down

4) letting your social supports in on your intention to change "I can't eat with you guys in the way I once did, but I still want to figure out a way we can connect"

5) creating a space in your home that signifies a new place to relax at the end of the day (so instead of on the couch with a bowl of chips, maybe it is a nice sheepskin rug with a beautiful chair, aromatherapy oils, and candles)

These are just some examples of a baptism that people have used in the past, but you may be cooking up something entirely different!

It must also be noted that you may have to return to your baptism several times throughout your life.

It is completely normal to have slips and relapses where you get off track. I think, psychologically, it is truly important to always go back to step 1 (baptism) when trying to get on track because each time you are symbolizing to yourself a new beginning.

If you are still unclear, think back to any time you have gotten off track with your diet for the first time and things were going so well. Didn't it seem like the next few times you tried to get back on track, it was never quite as good as the first time? That is in large part due to the fact that there is not as much pomp and circumstance around each attempt after the first one.

Here's another analogy (sorry I'm a sucker for a good analogy). It's like when you see the cars during Nascar races speeding furiously around the track, every once in a while they have to go off track to recalibrate. They have to take entire wheels off at times and put a new one on.

Don't you think they want to just hop right back out there so they can win the race? True professionals realize there is power in the beginnings of things, in going back to the drawing board. The Nascar recalibration and the baptism ritual of any addiction is no different.

Mind Meal: How will you recalibrate this time? What are some symbolic changes you could make in your life that would signify to you that this is the beginning of something major?

_____

_____

_____

_____

_____

_____

_____

_____

Chapter 8

Stop Waiting Until....

Many of us have a set of ideal values that we aspire to live by. We want to be healthy, kind, successful, spiritual, good, and the list goes on. However, in my practice, one observation I have made over and over is that everyone has their ideal version, and then there is a realistic version.

I always have wondered why people had such strong values, but their daily behaviors were not congruent with those values. For instance, some would really want to be a good parent, but they spent all their time at work and ruminating on the exhaustion and irritability that their children caused. Some had the value of "never getting a divorce," but continuously would hurl insults at their partners, ignore them, and put other priorities ahead of their marriage.

The same process takes place for many people struggling with food addiction. They strongly desire to lead a healthy and balanced life, yet when we peel apart their daily behaviors, nothing is congruent. They are forgetting to eat in the morning, rushing out the door, dealing with their busy days, until they become ravenous and go for yet another fast food or carb laden meal a co-worker orders to the office.

They don't want to succumb to hypertension, diabetes, chronic pain, sleep apnea, or any of the other myriad weight related complications their parents did. Yet, the continue to use food to cope with stress, loneliness, anger, and even to celebrate.

I began to realize that the narrative at the core of every person that sat in my office was "when _____ gets done, I will start _____." Everyone is waiting "until."

The problem is "until" rarely ever comes. Life throws a variety of things our way on a continual basis; illness, financial stress, death, loss, etc. If we always wait until the waters are calm- we may find ourselves in the golden years of our life resigning to let our deepest values go.

"Until" has to be right now. We have to begin to align our daily behaviors with our larger values. The saying "the days are long, but the years are short," implies that while we can get lost in the day to day- time flies, and we stand the risk of losing out on what we truly want for ourselves.

So how do I do this, you might ask? How do I align my days with my deepest held values?

It happens in baby steps.

Re-alignment with your deepest values doesn't happen overnight. We have to first identify what those are (which is a step many people haven't yet discovered). Then, we have to identify the behaviors that are congruent with that as well as the ones that are counterproductive.

We then plan out, realistically what that looks like in our day to day. For instance, if we identify daily exercise as something that is congruent with our value of being healthy and having longevity- then we may need to figure out how to restructure our day to accommodate for daily exercise.

If you realize that you are a night owl, and you have been trying to exercise in the morning before work- that would be a behavior that is not congruent, and more importantly- counter productive to your values. You would need to realize your personality and perhaps schedule exercise for the end of the day (vice versa for early birds).

Another exercise I use with clients is to have them sit down at the beginning of each morning and make 5-7 accomplish-able for the day. These might be the "fires" that need to be put out. The idea is that you narrow down what you are going to do TODAY, and then leave the rest for the next day.

When you finish these 5-7 accomplish-ables, you don't try and power through the rest of your list. Your goal then is to be present for that day. Go for a walk. Realign yourself with nature. Take a yoga class. Ask a friend to meet you for lunch. Call your mother. Watch a funny movie.

The idea behind this is that it allows us to feel like we are productive, we aren't checking out on life, bills get paid, kids get picked up from school, BUT we also focus on the present moment. This is a beautiful gift to ourselves and to our children.

Try it for one week. See how differently you feel as a result of focusing on being in the here and now. This will likely also translate into your eating behaviors. When we are present, we are less likely to be mindless and engage in grazing or mindless eating.

Mind Meal: What are three of your most deeply held values? What things have you used as an excuse to put off working on these values? What are the daily behaviors you could engage in that would start to realign you with your values again?

_____

_____

_____

_____

_____

_____

_____

Identifying
the
Obstacles

Chapter 9

Breaking the Cycle

You may find that you don't even realize when you eat. This mindless eating was born out of an emotional need originally. However, once we condition ourselves to engage in a behavior (eating) every time we experience a certain emotion, it becomes more and more of an unconscious process. Hence, the term "mindless" eating.

Your job is to now break the cycle and identify the key triggers that cause you to over eat. When I do evaluations, I often provide the client with four different types or styles of eating:

1. **the emotional eater** - the person who finds that certain (or all) emotions cause them to eat including ; boredom, stress, anxiety, loneliness, anger, happiness, etc.

2. **the skip & binger**- the person who fails to plan (and thus plans to fail) for food. They often skip breakfast,

even lunch, and don't eat until later in the day. They set up a feast or famine dynamic, over-indulging in too much food because they wait until the point they are ravenous to think about food. They often go for whatever is available, which is usually not whole, fresh, nutritious foods- but rather fast foods, or things that can sit on a shelf endlessly.

3. **the food addict**- the person who constantly thinks, obsesses about food. You could be eating a meal, and already planning for the next. At this point, food and the process of eating feels compulsive and almost out of your control.

4. **the miscellaneous** - this is a person who doesn't really identify with the other three categories, but overall they recognize they consume too large of portion sizes and eat the wrong types of food (unhealthy foods, junk foods, starchy carbs). This category or eating style is the one that usually has the most success with WLS because the surgery directly intervenes on the main issue (which is portion control).

Mind meal: Which of these categories do you fall into Do you find that you identify with multiple categories? What behaviors and thoughts lead you to believe you fall into these categories?

_____

_____

_____

_____

_____

_____

_____

Chapter 10

The Emotional Eater

This eating style is the second most worrisome for the psychologist because there are factors that contribute to weight gain that aren't fixed directly through WLS. If someone eats because they feel stress, they will still feel stress after the surgery- and are likely to continue to eat.

It's imperative that this behavior be nipped in the bud if you are to succeed with weight loss in the long term. Some people, unfortunately get the idea that they must just "white knuckle," the behavior to stop. In other words, when they would normally be triggered to eat, they just sit there saying over and over in their mind "don't eat, don't eat, don't eat," and we all know how well that works.

So instead, I encourage people to develop an alternative coping strategy that provides them with the benefit food once did. For example, if the person realizes that a big trigger for their emotional eating is to reduce boredom - my suggestion is to get a hobby.

If a person realizes they use food to demarcate the end of their work day and relieve stress- maybe they create a new ritual like making a really good cup of tea and curling up in their favorite blanket for 20 minutes.

If you notice that you use food as your "only justifiable break," because you work at home or you are a stay at home mom- the goal for you is to :

1) realize you need to justify another form of "break," for your health- it isn't selfish at this point and

2) figure out a different way to take a break such as going outside for a walk, calling a friend for a 10 minute chat, a 5 minute mindfulness of breath routine, adult coloring book, etc.

* Below is a sample tool I use with many clients to redefine how to deal with trigger emotions, that will inevitably still occur after weight loss.

Remedy

Trigger	Benefit of Food	Alternative Behavior
feeling tired	more energy	using lemon or peppermint essential oil
feeling lonely	feeling less lonely	reaching out to a friend or family member
sitting in front of tv	boredom reduced	adult coloring book, journal

Mind Meal: take a moment to make a list of all the associations, triggers, or emotional eating patterns you notice in your life.

The next step is to figure out the benefit of the food for each scenario (relaxation, stress relief, connection, reduced loneliness, anxiety relief, feeling of self care, feeling of being nurtured, etc).

The last step is to develop an alternative behavior that will give you the same benefit.

Triggers/Association: Benefits Alternative Behavior

_____ _____

_____

_____

Benefits:

_____

_____

_____

Alternative Healthy Behavior:

_____

_____

_____

Chapter 11

The Skip & Binger

They say if you fail to plan, plan to fail and this is certainly the case for the skip and binger type eater. This category is for those who don't necessarily feel they have an emotional attachment to food- but more that they fail to plan for food until it is too late. This eating style is one in which the person typically skips breakfast, maybe even lunch, and doesn't eat until much later in the day when they are RAVENOUS.

This obviously sets one up for failure because no one is in a good position to make good food choices when they are starving.

As a result, they tend to go for fast foods, vending machine snacks, or foods that can keep on shelves for years and thus aren't going to be super healthy for our bodies.

Through the years of working with the sporadic type eater, I've noticed they tend to consume most of their daily calories between 6 and 10 pm, the time of the day when we should be greatly decreasing what we put in our bodies before we shut it down for the night.

This unfortunately sets the person up for the same thing the next day. When they eat too late at night, they don't have natural hunger in the mornings, and thus the unhealthy cycle repeats itself.

I know it seems counterintuitive to think about food more to weigh less, but it's true. Those individuals who take an extra 1-2 hours of time at the beginning of the week to chop vegetables, clean produce and fruit, and at the least-put it in clear containers at eye level, are less likely to snack on unhealthy foods.

Additionally, those people that do a meal prep, either once a week, once a month, or once a day are less likely to indulge in unhealthy foods because they never get to the point of being ravenous.

Remedy

To remedy this unhealthy style of eating, try doing the following:

1) set alarms on your phone reminding you to eat in regular 2-3 hour intervals

2) engage in some form of meal prep (this can be once a day, once a week, or once a month)

3) invest in a nice big cooler to take with you throughout the day if you are a parent that is in the car a lot, a sales person, truck driver, or some other job that keeps you in a car for most of the day

4) Automation is key to eating healthy. If you are strapped for time and can't plan out every meal- at least create a list of meals and snacks you plan to make that week and use that as a guide for your grocery list. Here is an example:

– *tuna with olive oil, salt, pepper, on greens

– greek yogurt, granola, honey, and cinnamon

– pumpkin banana protein muffins

– roasted cauliflower with salmon

– protein shake with peanut butter and frozen

– bananas

– scrambled egg with feta and Sriracha

*this is a sample of my list, if you are undergoing WLS, please refer to your nutritionist for the specifics of what you can and can not eat

**Below are a small list of resources that you can use to help you plan ahead for meals throughout the week.

Resources

Pinterest is a great site to get healthy recipe ideas for free and you can even type in "vsg approved recipes" or "wls recipes," to get ideas.

Once a Month Meals, is a website that helps you to prep once a month, all of your meals, and this is by far the most cost effective method of meal prep (also the most time intensive).

Nowadays, there are some great meal delivery services that will meal plan for you and deliver all the fresh ingredients and spices right to your doorstep. For 6 meals- Blue Apron runs about $10/meal, which is a lot cheaper than Chinese take out or pizza (I've been using blue apron for 3 years, but also really like other brands). Plated, Home Chef, and Hello Fresh are also meal delivery options with comparable prices.

Amazon has great BPA free meal prep boxes too that come in a pack of 16 for around $19.99.

For a more complete guide to WLS resources including apps, books, and websites to make your journey easier, email me at talkdoc126@gmail.com for instructions on how to sign up for the online Full From Within Ultimate Course.

Mind Meal: What will be your way of planning? Meal prep on Sundays for the week? Once a month meal prepping? Will you use a delivery service? Can you foresee any conflicts or reasons why you would drop off- what safeguards could you put in place to ensure maintenance:

_____

_____

_____

_____

_____

_____

for a more comprehensive weight loss surgery resource guide be sure to check out my full from within course at schoolofselfhelp.teachable.com

Chapter 12

The Food Addict

The term "foodie," and "food addict" have become synonymous and sometimes interchangeable. Much like "chocaholic," the "food addict" term has lost its gravitas and seriousness.

When I say "food addiction," I am referring to someone with a long standing history of usually trauma and/or addiction to other things like drugs, alcohol, sex, or gambling. Food is usually the last "dragon that needs to be slayed."

You are likely to fall into this category if you have been through therapy for most of your life, diagnosed with multiple different mental health issues, struggled with addiction to other things, and likely experienced a heavy amount of physical and/or sexual trauma. This is the "level 3" referenced at the beginning of this book.

The food addict is also the one that usually needs the

gastric bypass surgery and has a significant amount of weight to lose (150+lbs). Unfortunately, they are often the ones who "slip through the cracks" during the pre-op eval process, get the surgery, and then develop dumping syndrome, regain the weight, and then come back a year later even more defeated than before.

If you feel you fall into this category, I strongly suggest that you find a therapist right away. Someone that specializes in trauma and eating disorders. The person you are working with should be able to provide psychoeducation about why we get cut off from our bodies when we experience trauma, thus making it difficult to ever feel full.

There are also a lot of additional trauma sequelae that effect one's weight. For instance, if someone experienced sexual assault, they may unconsciously try and build a cushion between themselves and the world around them. You can see how this make losing weight a complicated and painful process without the right trauma work.

If you identify as this type of eater- a "food addict," you fall into level 1, as mentioned in Chapter 2. Using the ocean levels analogy again, it would be difficult to just use this book to try and get your head above water. Not only are you stuck in the sand at the bottom of the ocean, but you have the weight of trauma holding you down.

It would be like saying "teach me to swim" all the while chained to a massive bag of bricks. You could learn to swim, but wouldn't it be easier to let go of that bag of bricks first?

This is what the right therapy can do. Notice, I say "the

right therapy," because just going to therapy once a week is not going to do it for severe trauma and addiction issues. Make sure to find the right therapist specialized and trained in trauma and eating disorders work.

To find referrals in your area, you can visit psychologytoday.com and type in your zip code and filter by insurance plan. You can also do this on goodtherapy.org.

One word to those that have already received the surgery and identify as being a food addict. All hope is not lost. The biggest step right now is identifying that there is a deeper problem and getting the necessary help immediately.

Mind Meal: Write down three therapeutic resources in your area that you could contact this week:

_____

_____

_____

_____

_____

_____

_____

Chapter 13

The Miscellaneous Eater

The miscellaneous category is the fourth category of eating style I present to pre-op patients when assessing the behaviors that got them into trouble in the first place. The miscellaneous type eater may not identify with any of the first three categories, but they just realize that overall - they consume too large of portion sizes (members of the "clean plate club") and often eat foods that are unhealthy and carb laden.

This type of eater is the easiest category to help and, in may opinion, the most successful with weight loss surgery. The reason being that 1/2 of their issue is immediately intervened with during gastric sleeve/bypass surgery. They are no longer able to clear their plate, and no matter how good a certain food tastes- they can only eat about the size of the palm of their hand at any one setting.

However, psychologically I do think it is still worth

addressing portion control. Many people who are getting WLS today, are members of the "clean plate club," because their generation grew up with parents that came out of the depression. Much of the zeitgeist at the time that current wls patients were children, was "waste not, want not."

For many of you, you feel guilty or wasteful when you see food being dumped in the trash, or going uneaten. To that I would say:

"would you rather have the food waste on your waist, or in the waste basket?"

Looking at it this way, often helps people to understand that once food is bought its going to "waste" somewhere. Our stomachs don't have to be the receptacles of allaying guilt anymore.

The other 1/2 of the miscellaneous eater's issue is selecting the wrong types of food. It could be that you feel your a "carb addict," a "chocoholic," have a "sweet tooth," or simply love salty, starchy foods.

I highly suggest you make use of the nutritionist consult required prior to all weight loss surgery. The nutritionist can be a wellspring of information about how to find recipes that satisfy certain cravings without sabotaging your plan.

Plus, a simple search of "weight loss surgery recipes" on amazon pulls up a list of books, chock full with recipes specifically tailored to post-operative guidelines. Pinterest is another great resource in terms of finding recipes that are healthy substitutions for cravings.

Many people secretly go into the surgery with the idea

that "I will still eat what I want, I just will eat less," and that will work initially. However, the problem is that it will catch up with you.

From a psychological standpoint, when we begin our day with junk, we are more likely to continue down that road.[10] Furthermore, we are less likely to go to the gym if we've been stuffing ourselves with junk food all day.

Mind Meal: How do you ensure that you avoid junk food for the most part in this next chapter of your life? What are some go to meals that you like, that are healthy, that could serve as "default" meals when you are busy:

_____

_____

_____

_____

_____

_____

_____

Chapter 14

Psychosocial Considerations during Weight Loss

One of the most common barriers for people after weight loss surgery is their social support system. When doing the pre-op evaluation, I always inquire as to who is living in the home, who have they told, and most importantly- are they supportive?

I have experienced many situations where the person's spouse is not on board and even skeptical of the procedure. This way of thinking becomes insidious to the relationship, especially after the surgery if there are side effects, difficulties with change, and/or complications. If the partner didn't feel the need for the procedure in the first place, it will be hard for them to be supportive afterwards.

This is why it is critical to sit down with your primary support system; spouse, girlfriend, boyfriend, sister, brother, parent, co-worker, boss- whomever you've chosen to tell, and make sure they understand the reasons you are doing this.

"The easy way out"

Many people are under the misinformed notion that this is "cheating," or "the easy way out." Ironically, once someone has been through post-op, they understand how misguided this is. Not only, do they have to do the same things everyone else has to do in terms of controlling their diet and exercising, but now they have to really limit their food to the things that won't wreak havoc later. There is no room for a cheat day in fact.

The first question I ask when doing a pre-op evaluation is "what has brought you to the point of considering this procedure?" Sometimes people will voice the frustration they've experienced trying on their own or yo-yo dieting throughout the years and they realize they need a power tool. Most of the time, people are facing life threatening diseases such as Diabetes, Hypertension, and Hyperlipidemia that are exacerbated by the weight they can't get off. They have family histories of moms and dads dying too soon and don't want to succumb to a similar fate.

Sometimes the reasons are even more unique. I had a man tell me that he traveled a lot for work and was humiliated every time they had to get him a seatbelt extender for the plane. I had a woman who said she wanted to finally be allowed to ride the rides with her kids at Knots Berry Farm.

These are the unique reasons that drive people to this procedure. It goes far beyond just wanting to look good poolside. This is what is imperative to explain to your support system.

I recommend taking a moment to write down all the reasons you are finally doing this. This becomes part of the conversation you have with your support system.

The conversation is not about asking permission but explaining clearly to them why you have decided on this. It is a time where they can express their concerns/fears, but not criticism.

If your hunch is that there may be some skepticism in your support system, the medical team can provide you resources to support the life saving benefits of weight loss surgery. Sometimes the numbers alone on medical tests after weight loss surgery, are enough to quiet most skeptics.

More importantly- YOU must become solid in the why. You must have clarity as to why you are doing this, or why you did this. If you are unsure- people will pick up on this and may sway you toward their own fears.

The next psychosocial consideration for weight loss surgery is post-operative support. Who will take you to your appointments? Who will run and pick up prescriptions for you if needed? Who will help meal plan with you?

The Dinner Table

The dinner table presents so many issues for so many. There are obviously a lot of cultures where food is the central gathering force. Many people find this the most difficult aspect post-operatively. Imagine your entire family sitting around for Sunday dinner, thanksgiving, or someone's birthday, you salivating over the french fries, birthday cake, or pizza, and everyone saying "come on, its just one day."

For some - this means removing themselves from the triggering environment all together. The conversation may look something like:

"I really love our time together at night when we can all get together for dinner, but I can't keep eating what you guys are eating if I really want to make this change. Being around for you guys longer feels better than anything on that table can taste and so I won't be at the dinner table anymore. But I still want to hang out. Could we all play cards afterwards? or could we go for a walk instead?"

This simple conversation, or a version of this- goes a long way in establishing a new way of relating to your family. It also helps establish accountability on your part because you are letting everyone know that you are changing significantly. It allays guilt of perceived loss of time with family. Lastly, it removes a major trigger that usually takes most people off course.

Mind Meal: What are the unique reasons you are doing this? Why is this so important to you?

_____

_____

_____

_____

_____

_____

_____

Filling You Back Up

Chapter 15

Repairing the self

What does it mean to be "full from within?" This concept refers to the idea that we no longer have this psychological "black hole," that needs to be fed through external things such as; food, drugs, alcohol, spending, relationships, gambling.

To be truly Full From Within means that our "tank" is mentally full. In other words, our self, although beaten up, bruised, and broken sometimes as a result of our journey down each of our unique life's path - is repaired and felt as whole again. Like a patchwork quilt that only gets stronger as a result of it's many tears and reparations.

How does one achieve this, you ask?

Borrowing from Aaron Beck's cognitive triangle [10]- we have three components of the mind that work to repair the self :

- thoughts

- feelings

- behaviors

These are the different components that must be running on all four cylinders to ensure that we aren't at risk of developing or perpetuating an unhealthy relationship with any of the topics mentioned above, for the purposes of this book, specifically - food.

Behaviors to Repair the Self

One of the biggest misconceptions about our mind is the idea that we must feel a certain way to engage in certain behaviors. In other words, we must first feel happy if we are going to go to a social event and relate to others in a positive way. However, the cognitive triangle mentioned above is tri-directional[14], meaning our behaviors can influence our feelings and/or thoughts, and vice versa.

This is powerful information. This means that we don't have to wait for happiness or joy to come around to engage in behaviors we know lend to more happiness. In fact, one of my first interventions with my patients who suffer from depression is the "just do it" approach, meaning they are given the task of doing three behaviors they don't necessarily feel like doing in the six days in between their next therapy session.

To explain depression via a very simple analogy- it is like the flu for the mind. What do you typically do when you have the flu?

You cancel your appointments, stay in bed, drink lots of water, and get lots of rest. The reasoning is that if we minimize the amount of life events for a brief bit of time, we will heal more quickly, and we do. BUT, this is not the case with depression.

The same intuition we use to combat the flu is the antithesis of what we must do to combat depression, yet somehow our instincts tell us to do the opposite. When we feel depressed, our inclination is to isolate, do less, and wait for the clouds to part. The problem with this, is that this type of behavior is what feeds the depression.

For my clients suffering with depression, I will often assign them a task of doing one social event, one bout of exercise (if they have never been inclined to exercise), and one learning activity (lecture, take a CE, attend a webinar, go to a pottery class, painting class, attend a speaking event).

Many of them balk at the idea. Some of them have been doing things their way for years and there is an undercurrent of fear related to breaking routine. It is almost as if the depression has a voice that says "don't do it, you will only feel worse."

I'm reminded of the saying "if you keep doing what you've always done, you'll keep getting what you've always got." Nothing could be more true when it comes to depression.

We must realize that when we have depression, our mind is sick. It is no longer serving us, and the messages are coming from crossed wires. In order to uncross those wires, we must physically and literally put one foot in front of the other and re-engage in those activities that we know from the research lend to a sense of happiness or at least contentment.

Below are some examples of behaviors, taken from my first book - Happiness in B.A.L.A.N.C.E : What We Know Now About Happiness [18.] :

- **Benevolence** - reaching out to others and getting out of our own head, focusing on how to make someone else's life or day better through connecting or giving

- **Play**- engaging in something that requires enough effort that we can't run old unhelpful tapes (I'm not good enough, other people must be more disciplined than me, things will never change, etc), but provides us with enough fun that we leave the activity feeling light, like surfing, artistry, building, writing, playing an instrument, etc.

  - When we are kids, we spend about 95% of our day playing and even trying to find play in our responsibilities (have you ever watched a kid brush their teeth or get dressed? it is never a straightforward buttoned up process). Yet, as adults - we flip that on its head and spend 95% of our time being a human doing vs. a human being.

- **Learning**- engaging in novelty is something our brain requires to feel happy and fed. It could be as simple as learning a new card game, all the way to enrolling in an MBA course. When we allow our minds to do what they are best at- our minds give back to us.

- **Connection**- We are social creatures by nature. There is a physiological rewiring process that occurs as result of being in near proximity to other humans [12]. It is how we survived so long ago, and our minds still provide the payoff.

- We are not meant to live in isolation, yet so many of us drift in this direction when they are depressed. Even introverts requires some social connection. While extroverts tend to thrive and recharge their batteries on social connection, it is true that introverts recharge in their solitude.

- However, there is a difference between being alone vs. lonely. As introverted as you may think you are, none of us are immune to going from alone to lonely if we don't make time for some social connection.

- **Exercise**- There are about 99 reasons to exercise and a happiness is one. I'm not going to waste space and wax poetic about the many benefits of exercise, because I'm sure you're well aware. But in addition to producing endorphins that have been proven to make us feel better, as far as weight loss goes- it also makes us less likely to put junk in our bodies. Ever do an intense sweat session and then make a beeline to the nearest McDonald's? I didn't think so.

Thoughts to Repair the Self

Mindfulness Based Cognitive Therapy is a 25 cent term to describe the process of looking at the old tapes we run in our minds day in and day out for years upon years, and stopping them in their tracks, and replacing them with new ones.

A hallmark approach in Byron Katie's book "Loving

What Is," is to continuously challenge one's thoughts by asking "is that really true?" [13] If we deem that we can't say with absolute certainty that a thought is true, then we can replace it with a more constructive thought.

For instance, if we find ourselves with a running narrative that goes something like "you are just never going to be someone that stands out, it's ok you have other good traits," then what is the behavior and feelings that it produces? Perhaps the person goes on feeling invisible like many people who are overweight feel. Maybe the person gives up on trying to stand out in the way they look and participate in life.

However, if we question that thought and say "can I know with absolute certainty that I will never stand out?" then the answer is "no." An alternative thought becomes, "I may have felt invisible leading up to this point, but there is no time like the present to make my mark. It is through my choices that I stayed in the shadows, but it will be through my new choices that will bring me back to life."

You can see how the latter alternative thought could bring forth a much different behavioral and feeling outcome. Is this hard work? Yes. Has anything worth getting in life ever come easy?

The good news is that the more we train the brain to think differently, the more differently we think, and the easier it becomes to think differently [16]. Recalling the tri-directional cognitive triangle mentioned above, thinking differently means behaving and feeling differently.

We have to curate our thoughts the way we curate our clothes. If we are mostly sad and hopeless in our lives, then we are bad dressers. We have to go into the closets of our minds and pull out the silkier more colorful thoughts.

Depression and anxiety are diseases of passivity, rendering us even more incapable of feelings of efficacy and internal control over our lives. However, it is only us that can pull us up from the depths of our despair by taking the reigns of this cognitive triangle by the horns.

Feelings to Repair the Self

The feeling component of the cognitive triangle is perhaps the most elusive. How do we make ourselves feel a feeling?

Research has shown that the simple behavior of smiling can induce a feeling of joy. So again the multi directional dynamic of the cognitive triangle is demonstrated. [17]

In fact, emotional pain like sadness and stress can be lessened through the act of smiling. If you are still skeptical about how our behaviors can change the tides of what often seem to be overwhelming emotional currents, try this exercise:

The next time you notice yourself feeling stressed or defeated when you get on the scale and notice it hasn't moved. Stop. Don't allow the mind to go down the well beaten path of beating yourself up.

Instead, immediately pull out photos of something that makes you happy, while playing upbeat or soothing music. You can go through a Digital album on Facebook or instagram, or even a physical album you have at home. Really focus on the details of those photos. Maybe it was a special trip you took with your mother, wife, or child.

Maybe it was the birth of one of your children. Maybe it was the day you bought your first house.

Notice how differently you feel? Doesn't it feel a little bit powerful to know how much we steer the ship when it comes to our feelings?

Additionally, we can influence our feelings by the thoughts we have. Obviously, if we have a running no-good narrative, playing on repeat, we aren't going to feel super awesome by the end of the day. But, if we start to employ Byron Katie's method of stopping and asking "do I know this to be absolutely true?" then we create room for change. An opportunity to feel differently and behave differently than we ever have before.

Mind Meal: Sit down and list the thoughts, feelings, and behavior triangles you believe to contribute to your unhealthy relationship with food. Try doing at least one that starts with your thought, one that starts with a behavior, and one that starts with a feeling.

Examples could be :

1. thought: I come from an overweight family, it's just our culture.

feeling: hopeless, defeated

behavior: Give up on trying to exercise or change eating patterns.

2. behavior: skipping the gym for two weeks

feeling: lethargic, tired, fatigued

thought: I don't feel like working out.

3. feeling: sad

thought: I don't want to be around anyone today.

behavior: skipping out on planned events with friends and family

Next, practice replacing the thought or behavior with a more silkier, colorful thought (recalling the clothes metaphor).

1. behavior: skipping the gym for two weeks

feeling: lethargic, tired, fatigued

thought: I don't feel like working out

Alternative behavior: making myself go to the gym

2. thought: I come from an overweight family, it's just our culture.

feeling: hopeless, defeated

behavior: Give up on trying to exercise or change eating patterns.

Alternative thought: It is time for me to finally break the cycle and be a positive role model for my parents and my children.

Use the space provided below to map out your cognitive triangles, and alternative thoughts:

_____

_____

_____

_____

Chapter 16

Mindfulness and weight loss

This might be one of my favorite topics to discuss with weight loss patients. Part and parcel of any addictive or habitual behavior is - mindlessness. Most people, at any given time, are ruminating in regret about the past, or fear of the future.

We condition ourselves to believe that the power to feel better lies in something outside of ourselves. However, just like Dorothy in the Wizard of Oz- it was always in your own back yard.

To cultivate mindfulness is a daily event. We must continuously be able to identify when we are caught up in an unhelpful "tape." You know the tape that tells us we aren't disciplined enough, the tape that rationalizes why today it is ok to not do our best, the tape that tells us the upcoming meeting is going to be rife with conflict and overwhelmingly stressful.

Simply identifying that a tape is playing is half the battle. Once we do this- we can take a step back and just observe the tape, without being swept up in it.

Another way to view mindfulness is to recall the telephone booths of the past. If we are inside the booth, it can be a torrential downpour all around us, yet we don't get wet. Mindfulness allows us to create this phone booth, this safe haven, by which to observe and accept the feelings instead of resisting them or being swept up in them.

When we practice mindfulness as it relates to our relationship with food, it might look like this:

You are standing in front of your pantry, looking for something to eat. You immediately snap to and question "what just happened right before this?"

Your response might be "oh yeah I just got a call that a bill is overdue and I am stressed now about our money this month. I went to food to help soothe me."

Instead you would take a step back. Close the pantry door. Sit and simply observe the anxiety or stress that might be present as a result of worrying about your financial situation.

The goal is not to judge the thoughts ("I need to relax. Other people don't stress this much") and simply observe and accept them. You can note how they are present in your body. Maybe you feel a tightness in your jaw, a warmth in your face?

Now, choose to focus on something else. Something that does not enhance the feeling of stress, but another feeling that is positive. Perhaps you open that funny email from a co-worker, maybe you go and read to your child or play a silly game, maybe you call your partner and plan a date night.

If you can build this muscle of bringing mindfulness to your mindlessness you will radically transform the way you relate to food.

Notice, not once did I mention that you meditate. People often confuse meditation with mindfulness. While mindfulness is a big part of meditation, I am speaking of a more general behavior that is applied throughout the day.

Meditation can also go a long way in reinforcing one's ability to be mindful. While the traditional prescription for meditation is usually 20 minutes X 2/ day, I realize that immediately sets some up for failure in that it is intimidating.

Instead, I encourage you to consider implementing the simple step of "beditation" by devoting the first 10-15 minutes of waking up with complete conscious silence. Don't hop on your phone, don't start talking to your partner- simply be. You may have to set your alarm to wake you up a bit early if you have a tight schedule in the morning, but I promise this will start to exponentially increase your ability to be mindful throughout the day.

Chapter 17

Happiness and weight loss

"Happiness is the meaning and purpose of life, the whole aim and end of human existence." –Aristotle

We know that weight loss can result in happiness, but did you know happiness can result in weight loss? As you probably already know being overweight can weigh on our ability to experience joy on a daily basis. Furthermore, many people are diagnosable at the clinical level for mild to moderate depression after being overweight for a long period of time.

The problem with depression is that it zaps us of our ability to do the very things that decrease depression (socialize, exercise, do novel things, create, etc). We feel unmotivated to do anything different than the day before, all the while telling ourselves, "eventually I'll get there." The problem is- that day never comes. If we keep doing what we've always done, we'll keep getting what we've always got.

Recovery from depression and/or cultivating happiness is literally about just doing it. Just doing it, despite the feeling that we so badly don't feel like doing it.

Today's view of happiness often connotes some sort of euphoric, blissful state. To some, happiness means an absence of all problems. This is a state that can not be realistically maintained. Life is constantly in a state of flux. Nothing is permanent. Happiness, or well-being is the ability and/or choice to experience peace in the presence of life's ups and downs.

Many of us experience anxiety or worry on a daily basis. This feeling was once a survival mechanism. If we remained hyper-vigilant, we were less likely to be eaten by a lion or tiger. However, in today's modern society- those lion and tigers no longer exist. They have taken the form of bills to pay, jobs to complete, and relationships to repair.

The problem is that these modern day worries are no where close to the problems we once faced (literally being eaten alive by an animal or any of the hundreds of other dangers that existed in our early ancestry). Yet, our brain does not differentiate. So it is upon us, along with the help of our nifty relatively new frontal cortex to put things in perspective.

Case Example: A client came in the other day and was complaining of always being "on," and not being able to turn off. She talked about her neighbor's dog, who kept going in her grass.

She talked about her need to wave to all the neighbors in the neighborhood as she drove by. She was genuinely upset at her inability to shut off.

I jumped to a completely different topic, one about a story I heard on NPR about a small Ukranian village, where the children were starving and couldn't get access to fresh water or vaccines. I related it to us in our current lives. We will never face the issue of starvation. We will always have access to clean water, and modern medicine.

Immediately, her "lion" was put into perspective. At the end of the session, I encouraged her to "look down" instead of "up" if she was going to engage in the bad habit of comparison.

We can all take a page off this example. Whenever we get mired in the day to day, ask yourself "will this matter in five years." If the answer is no, do something to distract your mind, and move on.

So now that we have a good starting point of what NOT to do, what should we do to ensure our happiness is nourished and cultivated?

In my book, Happiness in B.A.L.A.N.C.E: What We Know Now [23], I created a seven factor model, based on the happiness research. These seven factors can easily be remembered by the acronym BALANCE. I did this on purpose so that the reader or client has an easy way of checking in with themselves and making sure they are doing all they can to experience well being.

Below, I will outline the seven factors of happiness,

according to current research in evolutionary psychology. If you want a more thorough explanation, or want to know how better to apply it to your life, please check out the book, which can be found on my website or amazon.com:

Benevolence- also referred to as altruism, benevolence is a key behavior that fosters a feeling of connection, value, and purpose. Research has demonstrated that acts of benevolence actually stimulate the pleasure centers of the brain.[19]

Awareness- awareness, in this case, refers to the conscious thought processes. It includes our ability to navigate social situations, negotiate conflict, and to avoid discord. Awareness was a significant factor in enabling our species to get along and collaborate with fellow tribes.

Without this awareness, we are pinged back and forth throughout our life, like a pinball machine, without a clue as to why things "never go our way."

Learning- this includes both challenge and purpose. It is the behavior of the lifelong learner. This factor helped our species to remember predatory areas, locations for sustenance, and which people belonged to your family. We are hardwired as humans to continuously learn, and when we don't- our psyches pay the price.

Active Flow- The term "flow" was first coined by Mihaly Csikzentmilhalyi [20] and referred to the simultaneous convergence of heightened engagement and optimal performance. Think back to a time hen you were completely immersed in something. This could be whilst playing tennis, surfing, or painting a picture. Active flow allows us to turn down the volume on that anxious part of the brain and engage in something that is uniquely suited to our own individual talents.

Active flow acts as a sort of neurological dam, providing our minds sanctuary form the harsh internal climate of our brain. This flow probably helped early man too- think of what the current state of affairs might be if they had not painted, created language, symbols, or tools.

Nurturing Relationships- It doesn't take a rocket scientist to tell you about the importance of relationships to the human race. It is blatantly obvious how relationships are directly connected to our ability to survive and reproduce. Ironically, most everyone can understand how vital relationships are, yet many spend very little time investing and cultivating in them, especially when we feel bad about our outside appearance.

Calming meditation- religious ritual is on the of the few behaviors that separate us from the animals. Archaeological studies demonstrate that religious ceremonies have been performed since the beginning of man.[26] There is something innate within all of us which drives us to look in wonderment at the sky above us and ponder whats out there.

Research has shown key areas of the brain, associated with well being, to be intensely active within individual who are in deep prayer or meditation.[22] Meditation also helps to regulate that nasty hormone cortisol, that is partly responsible for a pillowy gut. [23]

Exercise, nutrition, & sleep- If meditation is the screwdriver that builds our happiness, exercise is the power drill. In his groundbreaking book, Why Zebras Don't Get Ulcers, Robert Sapolsky[24] posits that our bodies aren't designed to handle the long term stress of sitting in traffic jams and growing up in poverty, they have been developed more for the short term stress a zebra might face.

Of course, when faced with a threat, a zebra would immediately run, thereby reducing the stress. It makes sense that running is now one of the most effective methods for decreasing cortisol, and ultimately our own stress.

Nutrition falls under this umbrella (sorry couldn't fit another "n" in balance). Most of you think about nutrition in a caloric sense, but there is significant research that evidences the types of food we consume have a strong influence over how we feel. [25]

Finally the last piece that falls under the "E" is sleep (again acronym struggled a bit, but you get the idea). Sleep is a lot like sex. If we are getting enough of it, it's about 2% on our priority ladder. If we aren't getting enough of it, its about 99%. Sleep is a significant factor in the happiness equation.

Research also has found a connection to greater amounts of sleep and less abdominal fat. [26] So the next time, your partner gets on you about going to bed early, or sleeping in- say "I'm working on my abs."

Chapter 18

Your Power Tools

So here is where the rubber really meets the road in terms of where this book can help you make some concrete changes in your lifestyle. The following tools are tools I have used with my weight loss clients for the last 10 years in private practice. These are the tools that I encourage each person to develop on their own so that they become personally meaningful and motivating.

For instance, I could guess that a mom might want to lose weight to keep up with her young kids, but when she says "I want to be able to ride the rides with them at Knotts berry farm," I know that is something personally meaningful to her, that will power her through those urges.

Take a look at the tools that follow and develop your own based on the examples. You can create them using the canva app, very easily, you can make individual lists in your phone, or physically make them and laminate them.

The Cons List

A powerful tool to give you a boost in motivation to change is to take a moment to list all of the reasons you want to dramatically change your relationship with food. Having this tool close by, will serve you well in the midst of emotional triggers and cravings.

- Eating sugar and carb laden food leads to wanting more of it

- guilt about eating unhealthily and not being strong enough to stop

- Not fitting into clothes

- Wanting to isolate and hide because you have a poor self image

- Weight gain

- Low self-esteem

- Losing confidence professionally and socially

- Feeling bloated, nauseated, or listless

The Happy List

HAPPY LIST

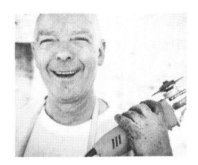

MOVIE SOUNDTRACK STATION
SITTING ON FRONT PORCH
TAKING A SPIN CLASS
FIXING SOMETHING
PLAYING CARDS WOTH FRIENDS
GAMES WITH KIDS
DOG WALK
WATCHING A FUNNY MOVIE
SHOPPING
PLANNING A TRIP
EXPLORING A NEW PLACE
HIKING
READING A BOOK
TAKING A LONG BATH
GETTING A MASSAGE

The tool to help one shift how they define quality of life starts with the "happy list," and it is simply what it says on the tin- a list of things that uniquely bring YOU happiness outside of food.

The idea behind this tool is to help you define quality of life and enjoyment by things outside of eating. If going out to eat or having a starchy carb-laden dinner is the thing you're living for each day, every day after surgery (or during your diet) is going to feel like deprivation or like you're putting your real life on hold. Let's admit it- no one will put themselves through anything they perceive as deprivation for too long, that's why most diets fail.

What's on YOUR happy list? Feel free to comment on our private Facebook page to give others inspiration.

Triggers

These are all the pesky little buggers that cause us to do the very things we say we don't want to do anymore. For some, it is simply 5 pm rolling around and wanting to demarcate the end of the day. For others, a trigger might be an in-law who is overly critical and causes them to self soothe through food. Another trigger can be as simple as an emotion that comes up like boredom or stress.

Shining the light of our consciousness on these triggers no longer allows them to perpetrate in the way they once did. It is easy to call out the main ones, but it is important to take some time and really do a full mental inventory of all the triggers that can cause you to relapse. Maybe it's a county fair? Maybe its those weekly co-worker birthdays? Maybe it is the ritual of having a "secret" and eating when no one is around.

Take some time to investigate all the people, emotions, thoughts, events, and behaviors that can trigger an eating episode for you.

Coping Strategies

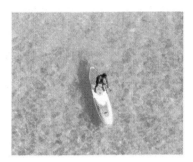

COPING SKILLS

ADULT COLORING
CALL MY SISTER
TAKE A HOT BATH
GO FOR A WALK
ORGANIZE
PAINT MY NAILS
WORK ON MOTORCYCLE
CREST WHITE STRIPS
MEDITATE
MAKE A PLAYLIST
CHECK EMAIL
CARE FOR A PET
GO TO A MEETING
ONLINE SUPPORT FORUM
JOURNAL
WORKOUT APP
PHYSICAL THERAPY
PINTEREST/FACEBOOK

Take a few moments to map out what your coping strategies will be. You can use the template I have included above, or just make your own. I suggest keeping it on you or in your phone so that you will have immediate access at all times.

To create a visually appealing coping strategy list such as the one above:

- download the canva app for free
- pick an image that inspires you (free high res images on unsplash.com)
- and select a template, and simply type in your coping strategies
- If you feel you are less "tech savvy," it is ok for you to just write them down on a piece of paper, your journal, or a list in your phone.

Why do we need coping strategies? The rule of the brain is what fires together, wires together- so if you pair food with stress, or food with 5pm when you walk in the door, or food when your laying on the couch at night- you soon unconsciously eat because the wiring has been so strongly reinforced. The idea is to clip the wire and begin to pair the triggers and associations with alternative coping skills.

From the addiction research, we know that a craving lasts 3-5 minutes.[27] So the idea is to watch the addicted midbrain rise and fall like a wave, yet not be swept up by it. During that craving we simply sit back psychologically and observe the mind like "isn't that interesting how many times my addicted mind has told me that food would be a good idea right now, but I don't have to listen to it now- I can tell myself a different story."

It usually takes around one to three months to start noticing true change taking place, so don't get frustrated with your self if you slip or have an off day.

Spirituality

If you recall an earlier part of this book, I mentioned that the two pillars of all recovery from addiction are healthy interpersonal relationships and spirituality.

Spirituality is a tough one. For many, it connotes religion. It brings the thought of a dogmatic set of do's and don'ts.

To clarify, spirituality is different for everyone, but let me be clear- it is essential for everyone. It is the thing that anchors us back to our souls. It reconnects us with ourselves, others, a higher power, a sense of purpose and meaning, and it prevents us from isolation.

I once read "religion is what gets you into heaven, but spirituality is what brings you out of hell." Spirituality can encompass a myriad of different things for each person, but it is a pillar of addiction recovery in almost all modes of treatment. Below are some examples of how one might start cultivating the spiritual:

- going for nature walks
- being of service to someone or the community
- meditation or prayer
- going to a meeting of other spiritual people and learning different beliefs and finding the ones that resonate with you
- paying gratitude each day
- Playing or giving back to one's self
- devoting time to something higher than one's self
- acting with principle and integrity even when no one is watching

If we can connect with the light that exists within all of us, we get even closer to facing the darkest parts of ourselves and exposing our own psychological parasites.

My New Self Vision

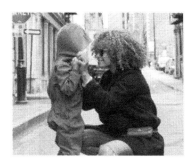

Another important visual tool to put in your arsenal of change, is the "my new self vision," tool. This can be, again, another list you write in your journal, in your phone, or somewhere on your fridge. It can also be something you create such as the one above, laminate, and keep as part of your visual tool belt.

To create one like the picture above, you can follow the steps for canva I outlined in the "emotional eater" chapter.

Your self vision can be composed of people or aspects of people you want to cultivate yourself. Ever heard the expression "be the change you want to see in the world"?

Alternative Idea: The Vision Board

I want you to get a large piece of poster board and a stack

of magazines. Dedicate about an hour of your time to going through the magazines and clipping pictures of items and people that represent how you'd like to look or feel after you've met your goals.

This could a yoga model that looks healthy and at peace, a bottle of smart water to represent always being hydrated, a father with his kids to represent a renewed sense of vigor, a tropical island to represent how you will start rewarding yourself and spending your new found time (guess what-food addiction takes up a lot of unnecessary time).

Once this has been constructed, ideally you should put it in a place you will see every day and can meditate on. If space is limited, you can take a picture with your phone and set it as your wallpaper. The idea is to utilize the powers of intention and attraction to bring forth your vision for yourself.

My Dailies

This tool is comprised of all the things you know you need to do on a daily basis to keep you on the straight and narrow. I love this list, especially for people who have any notion that weight loss surgery is "the easy way out." When you actually take a look at all the things you have to juggle on the daily, it becomes resoundingly clear, this is not a cake walk.

Think about all the things that you know you will need to do to comply with post-op instructions as well as the behaviors that will signify to you- that today is a new day.

Below is an example of one client's dailies:

- wake up- first 10 minutes meditate and set daily intention

- Write in journal

- write down three things I am grateful for today

- take vitamins

- drink hot lemon water

- meal prep for the day

- do yoga online or go for a run

- reach out to one person to check on them

- one "bank deposit" (self care item)

Mind Meal: Take some time (about an hour) to make these tools for yourself. It can be as simple as writing down on a piece of paper, making a word doc, or putting lists in your phone. You want to make sure that these lists/tools are always close by.

Closing

So what does it all mean? Can we truly be full from within? If I've done my job in this book, you should be left with a sense that it is not any one thing that fills us up, but a balance of many things at the same time.

To be full from within, we must rid our inner selves of

the toxicity that resulted in our unhealthy relationship with food in the first place, and then continuously fill ourselves back up with the things that go into making us feel "full."

This does not happen overnight, and we are never done. It is a continual process that occurs throughout our lives that must be maintained.

I'll leave you with one of my favorite metaphors. That of the bonsai tree:

Bonsai trees are fantastic plants. They are not genetically predestined to be dwarfed. In fact, they can be created from visually any plant. It is the technique of cultivating, potting, pruning, and shaping that determines their outcome. Improper pruning can weaken, or even kill the tree.

Similarly, our ability to be truly "full from within" is not genetically predetermined. Although some expression of our genes will ultimately be revealed, it is our continuos shaping, pruning, and cultivating that will influence what the final outcome looks like.

With enough care and attention aimed towards our "fullness," we will survive and thrive this life. We will finally develop a healthy relationship with food.

However improper treatment can also lead to our detriment. It is through a balance of behaviors that we finally understand how to become full from within...

References

[1] Bergland, C. (2014, March 20). New Clues on the Inner Workings of the Unconscious Mind. Retrieved May 7th, 2017, from https://www.psychologytoday.com/blog/the-athletes-way/201403/new-clues-the-inner-workings-the-unconscious-mind

[2] Bergland, C. (2014, March 20). New Clues on the Inner Workings of the Unconscious Mind. Retrieved May 7th, 2017, from https://www.psychologytoday.com/blog/the-athletes-way/201403/new-clues-the-inner-workings-the-unconscious-mind

[3] www.garylangephd.com/userfiles/4688565/file/AddictionBrainLtHd.doc

[4] Carey, B. (2007, July 31). Who's Minding the Mind? The New York Times. Retrieved from http://www.nytimes.com/2007/07/31/health/psychology/31subl.html?pagewanted=all&_r=0

[5] The Conscious, Subconscious, And Unconscious Mind - How Does It All Work? (2014, March 13). Retrieved May 7th, 2017, from http://themindunleashed.org/2014/03/conscious-subconscious-unconscious-mind-work.html

[6] NeuroScience Technical Bulletin, 2010, "Glutamate and Addiction, Issue 29; www.neurorelief.com

[7] McCauley, Kevin, 2009, "Pleasure Unwoven" DVD, Institute for Addiction Study

[8] Sinacola, R., and Peters-Strickland, T. (2006). Basic psychopharmacology for counselors and psychotherapists. Boston: Allyn and Bacon

[9] http://communicate.eckharttolle.com/news/2014/08/13/when-the-pain-body-awakens/

[10] https://www.sciencealert.com/eating-junk-food-triggers-a-cycle-of-unhealthy-food-choices

[11] Carr, A. (2005) Easy way to stop drinking. Sterling.

[12] Cognitive Therapy and the Emotional Disorders , Aaron T Beck 1976, penguin group

[13] Katie, B., Mitchell, S. (2002) Loving what is : Four questions that can change your life. New York. Harmony books.

[14] Depression-related cognitions: antecedent or consequence?. Journal of abnormal psychology, 90(3), 213.

[15] Lyons, L. C., & Woods, P. J. (1991). The efficacy of rational-emotive therapy: A quantitative review of the outcome research. Clinical Psychology Review, 11(4), 357-369.

[16] Rimm, D. C., & Litvak, S. B. (1969). Self-verbalization and emotional arousal. Journal of Abnormal Psychology, 74(2), 181.

[17] https://www.ncbi.nlm.nih.gov/pubmed/7381683

[18] Long, C. (2010) Happiness in balance: what we know now. California. Createspace

[19] http://www.wildmind.org/blogs/news/altruism-hard-wired-to-pleasure-centers-in-brain

[20] https://en.wikipedia.org/wiki/Flow_(psychology)

[21] http://www.ancient.eu/religion/

[22] https://www.scientificamerican.com/article/the-neurobiology-of-bliss-sacred-and-profane/

[23] https://www.ncbi.nlm.nih.gov/pubmed/23724462

[24] Sapolsky,R. (2004) Why Zebras Don't Get Ulcers. Macmillan

[25] http://www.health.harvard.edu/blog/nutritional-psychiatry-your-

brain-on-food-201511168626

[26] https://sleepfoundation.org/sleep-news/sleep-linked-gains-abdominal-fat

[27] Retrieved May 29, 2017 http://www.everydayhealth.com/hs/quit-smoking/ways-snuff-cigarette-cravings/

[28] Retrieved: June 2, 2017
https://www.madinamerica.com/author/rwhitaker/

50594744R00060

Made in the USA
San Bernardino, CA
27 June 2017